Fitness of the Future: Getting Started With Fitness Technology

J. Steele

Published by RWG Publishing, 2023.

While every precaution has been taken in the preparation of this book, the publisher assumes no responsibility for errors or omissions, or for damages resulting from the use of the information contained herein.

FITNESS OF THE FUTURE: GETTING STARTED WITH FITNESS TECHNOLOGY

First edition. January 18, 2023.

Copyright © 2023 J. Steele.

Written by J. Steele.

Also by J. Steele

Gemstone Guide Book: A Simple Informative Handbook
Born to Win: Discover Unlimited Possibilities
Think You Can and You Will: How to Become a Champion in Life
Quick and Easy Guide on Dieting
Quick and Easy Guide on Fashion
Alcohol and Addictions
Online Dating
Lose Weight Dieting
Lose Weight Fasting
Ways To Lose Weight For Women
Raw Food and Healthy Living
Back Pain Recovery Informative Guide
100 Health Suggestions: A Healthy Lifestyle is Beneficial to the Soul
Tips for Bodybuilding
Vegetarianism's Advantages
Fitness of the Future: Getting Started With Fitness Technology
The Shadow's Blade: A Tale of Magic and Betrayal

Table of Contents

Introduction - Why do we need fitness? 1

Chapter 1 – What Exactly is Wearable Technology? should I use it 5

Chapter 2 – The evolution and history of wearables 9

Chapter 3 - Different Types of Wearable Technologies and Are They Safe? 13

Chapter 4 - Advantages of using technology over not using it 17

Chapter 5 - Things to consider before investing 19

Chapter 6 - A comparison of wearable technologies and smartphone applications 23

Chapter 7 - Avoiding Common Wearable Technology Newbie Mistakes 25

Chapter 8 – Integrating wearable technology into everyday life 29

Conclusion - The future of wearable technology: where did it come from here? 33

Introduction - Why do we need fitness?

Welcome to our beginner's guide to the future of fitness technology and wearables. I just want to thank you for joining me as we embark on this rapid journey of discovery in this ever-changing landscape of technological advancement. In this first introductory chapter, we look at why we need fitness and how technology plays/will play a major role in keeping us fit. Let's get started...

First and foremost, we live in an era where high-fat fast food is available on every corner and advertised on every available platform. No wonder more and more people are overweight. Obesity in the dictionary is defined as

"The condition of being very fat or overweight; obesity."

There are dire consequences for those who are morbidly obese. Check out the facts and figures on obesity around the world...

According to the World Health Organization (WHO), global obesity rates doubled between 1980 and 2008. In 2014, 39% of adults aged 18 and over worldwide were overweight (approximately 2 billion), of whom 19% were considered obese (about 1 billion). People).

The statistics for childhood obesity are equally alarming. WHO revealed that the number of overweight and obese children under the age of five increased to 41 million from 31 million in 1990.

How is obesity measured?

It is measured using BMI or body mass index. This can be calculated by taking a person's weight in kg and dividing it by their height in meters. Note that this does not differentiate muscle-related weight from the fat-related weight. Therefore, with this in mind, BMI provides an unpredictable measure of fat. BMI is therefore considered a "rough guide" because it does not correspond to the same level of obesity in everyone.

A person who has a BMI over 25 is "overweight". However, if someone has a BMI of 30, they are considered obese.

Obesity is the leading cause of preventable death. A child or adult with clinical obesity is at risk of high cholesterol, high blood pressure, heart disease, stroke, type 2 diabetes, joint problems, cancer, depression, and respiratory problems.

Perhaps the light behind all these grim facts is that obesity can be reversed... especially with the help of fitness technology!

In contrast to people who suffer from other diseases, children or adults who are obese can fight obesity by prioritizing health and fitness.

it's too late If you or someone you know is obese, here are 5 key ways to reverse its effects:

1) Eliminate Sugar, Salt, and Saturated Fat - High intake of salt, sugar, and saturated fat contributes to obesity. WHO has

reduced the recommended intake of fat (53 g/day), sugar (25 g/day), and salt (5 g/day) to reduce the risk of diabetes and obesity in the global population.

2) Adequate sleep and managing stress - Sleep deprivation and chronic stress are major causes of insulin imbalance and weight gain. Poor sleep patterns are linked to metabolic disturbances and increased cravings for carbohydrates and sugar. Religious adherence to at least 8 hours of uninterrupted sleep combined with activities that promote relaxation (yoga, meditation, massage, etc.) can help reverse the effects of type 2 diabetes.

3) Educate yourself about nutrition - Food is the body's fuel, allowing us to think and do everyday tasks, but it is important to be careful when choosing food. Except for maintenance WHO recommends an intake of fat, sugar, and salt, adding whole, unprocessed foods (such as vegetables, fruits, and nuts) to the diet can prevent insulin resistance and in turn help reverse obesity. The right set of multivitamins and supplements can also promote proper fat and sugar metabolism. If you are unsure about the proper diet and supplements, it is best to seek advice from a nutritionist.

4) Exercise - Any physical activity, whether walking for a few hours or doing 30 minutes of high-intensity interval training, is better than nothing. Make sure you get your heart rate up when you exercise.

5) Measure Progress - Many studies show that people who track their diet and exercise progress with a notebook or chart lose twice as much weight. Self-monitoring is a tedious task, as BMI

readings, calorie intake, and physical activity are recorded manually, but fitness phone apps make it a lot easier. With fitness trackers that can track everything from steps, distance walked, pace, estimated calories burned, and even sleep patterns, self-monitoring offers more motivation than ever before.

Anyone diagnosed with obesity may or may not perceive the situation as grim. Lifestyle, diet, and fitness changes can help prevent or reverse the effects of obesity, and with the help of fitness technology, fighting obesity is easier than ever!

Well, this is a basic introduction to the current obesity situation in the world and why we need fitness and health. In the next few chapters, we'll take a closer look at what wearable technology is, how it can help with fitness, and how it can affect you. Are you ready? Let's go...

Chapter 1 – What Exactly is Wearable Technology? should I use it

First, we have to ask ourselves the question... what exactly is wearable technology? Wearable technology, short for wearable technology, are gadgets or devices that are worn on the body along with clothing and other accessories to help users perform various functions that can be performed on computers and mobile phones while on the move.

These gadgets usually contain some sort of tracking technology (e.g. motion sensors) that monitor various data such as heart rate, sleep pattern, physical activity (steps, productivity, etc.), and various other useful information.

Wearable technology has many uses and can benefit people of all ages who suffer from:

* Obesity – The biggest industry that wearables have infiltrated is health and wellness. Today you can find bracelets, sports bras, jewelry, watches, belts, and other items programmed to monitor physical activity, function as pedometers, offer workouts, measure intake and calories burned, and track other bodily functions.

Popular wearable fitness trackers such as FitBit and JawBone have helped users motivate themselves through exercise. Meanwhile, overweight kids can make weight loss fun with a variety of portable play equipment that encourages activity, provide challenges, and allow them to play against other kids.

*Insomnia and Sleep Apnea – Sleep is an important part of fitness, so wearable devices that monitor a person's sleep quality can be very helpful. Neuro: On, Luciding, ActiGraph, Fatigue Science RediBand, FraSen Inc. Sleep Mask, and Sleep Image are tools with a comprehensive list of sleep data analytics that can help people with insomnia and sleep apnea.

Fitness trackers like the Garmin VivoSmart and the UP3 from Jawbone that come with a sleep monitor are great for users who also want to prioritize their health. The Kokoon in-ear sleep headphones are said to improve people's sleep, but they won't hit the market until late 2016.

* Age-related diseases – Older people who suffer from age-related diseases such as cataracts, diabetes, high blood pressure, arthritis, and cardiovascular disease (among others) may also find wearables very useful. For example, BodyGuardian sensors can perform cardiac EKG and rhythm monitoring on patients and provide the results to the respective doctor.

* Back problems – Devices like UPRIGHT and Lumo Lift remind people of posture, which is the number one cause of unnecessary back pain. Valedo strengthens muscles to prevent back pain, while Cur claims to use electrical stimulation to relieve back pain at its source.

* Asthma – Health Care Originals developed Smart Asthma Management, a wearable that aids symptom recognition,

FITNESS OF THE FUTURE: GETTING STARTED WITH FITNESS TECHNOLOGY

medical treatment plan reminders, and other asthma management features.

* Diabetes – Google Life Sciences has launched an ambitious project that could potentially help reverse the effects of diabetes. Truly a contact lens that detects glucose levels.

Wearable technology can also benefit people who are perfectly healthy but want to improve their performance through sports, exercise, and strength training in addition to other physical activities.

Sports fans are going crazy for wearables that can provide real-time game statistics and accurate measurements of player performance.

In some cases, wearable technology can help save lives, encourage healthier lifestyles and prevent disease.

Chapter 2 – The evolution and history of wearables

Wearable technology may be all the rage in 2016, but the process of incorporating technology into everyday life has been going on for centuries. According to Giordano da Rivalto, the earliest "smart glasses" were commissioned by the Roman Emperor Nero. The glasses consist of a metal frame and emerald green lenses, which are said to have helped improve Nero's eyesight during the battles of AD 54–68.

In the 17th century China, the oldest smart ring was designed using the smallest abacus you will ever see.

In 1884, Cute Circuit's Electric Girls demonstrated one of the first uses of wearables in New York fashion. The electric light is embedded in a bunch of ballet flats.

In 1907 Julius Neubronner in Germany invented the first GoPro-like device and sub-niche of pigeon photography. He attaches several pigeons to an aluminum chest strap holding a miniature self-timer camera that takes a single aerial photo.

In the early 1960s, the term wearable technology had not yet been coined but had been applied to countless inventions. Two MIT professors, Edward Thorpe and Claude Shannon, designed, built, and tested the world's first portable computer capable of predicting the outcome of roulette. The device consists of two main parts - a timer hidden inside the shoe and a cigarette case. Thorpe and Shannon were so successful that their winning bet rose to 44% and led to the passage of the Nevada law in 1985 outlawing such machines.

Also in the 1960s, the earliest HUDs (head-up displays) and wearable virtual reality devices were developed by a single person. In 1960, cinematographer Morton Heilig invented a large chest-worn device called the Stereophonic Head-Mounted Television Screen (HMD) that combined his love of cinema with virtual reality. Two years later, he patented a 4DX VR simulator-like device he dubbed the "Sensorama Simulator", which consisted of a vibrating chair, stereo speakers, a steering wheel, special effects such as an air blower, and headphones that produced a particular smell in the game. location movie

During the last quarter of 1975, Pulsar sold 100 limited editions "watch calculators" made of 18 ct gold and priced at $3,950.

In July 1979, Sony launched the brand's historic Walkman, the first portable cassette player.

A high school student named Steve Mann developed the first backpack computer with a headset-mounted CRT camera viewfinder in the early 1980s. Mann invented and pioneered many wearable technologies related to photography, such as the first handheld wireless webcam in 1994.

X-Games owes much to mountain biker Mark Schulze, who attached a video camera to his helmet, and produced an instructional video in 1988 entitled "The Great Mountain Biking Video" which is viewed on YouTube by many GoPro fans.

FITNESS OF THE FUTURE: GETTING STARTED WITH FITNESS TECHNOLOGY

Tons of wearable technology has emerged since the 2000s, from Bluetooth headsets to 100% Vitatron C-Series digital pacemakers. The explosion of wearable fitness devices can be traced back to the Nike and Apple collaboration on the iPod fitness tracker, which inspired the first wearable fitness gadget FitBit. In 2012, one of the most popular Kickstarter success stories was The Pebble's customizable smartwatch after the founders raised over $10 million.

When Google Glass was introduced in 2013, the rest is history. From now on, every brand from mobile, fitness, IT, sports, entertainment, and more wants to bring wearables to the market, that's why 2014 is called "The Year of Wearable Devices".

Chapter 3 - Different Types of Wearable Technologies and Are They Safe?

In this chapter, we look at some of the wearable technologies expected to conquer the technology industry as the need for smaller portable computers grows, and whether or not they are safe to use.

Wearable smart glasses

These are glasses with an embedded microchip that are worn on the face to help the user perform several tasks without realizing it. It can help take pictures, record videos, magnify objects, improve eyesight, and can be used as industrial detection glasses.

There are several wearable smart glasses that are trending lately, including Google Glass, Vuzix M100, Recon Jet, GlassUp, Meta Pro, Epson, and Moverio.

smartwatch

A smartwatch is a wrist-worn device with a touchscreen display that connects to your smartphone via Bluetooth and keeps you up to date with your phone's digital network, e.g. B. Notifications for incoming calls, emails, and various app notifications about who you work with, tracking daily activity, and more.

Some of the most talked about smartwatches on the market today are the Apple Watch, TAG Heuer Smartwatch, Pebble Time, and others.

fitness tracker.

This is a great bracelet or watch made to help you track and quantify your fitness activities. They tell you how far you walked or ran, how many calories you burned, when you didn't sit properly, how many calories you burned, track your heart rate, and more. They usually come in a variety of styles, shapes, colors, and sizes.

Smart clothes

This is a garment with small, built-in sensors designed to monitor and provide feedback on your health, fitness, and athletic activity. They are also worn by the military on the front lines of war to provide soldiers with some form of health and emergency care when injured or in danger. These clothes are usually stiff and heavy and cannot be worn under normal circumstances. In recent years, there have been innovations in smart wear that are more fashionable and comfortable.

Recent smart wearers include Google's Project Jacquard, Athos; Medical-technical clothing for fitness studios. Mbody Bike & Run for runners and cyclists. Sensoria running socks; are used to track walking time, distance, and pace. Elegant Synapse Dress; that gives a blue light signal when someone approaches, B is in labor; Climachill Health Tracker Maternity Dress by Adidas; Used to make the wearer feel cold when running.

FITNESS OF THE FUTURE: GETTING STARTED WITH FITNESS TECHNOLOGY

Smart jewelry

Smart jewelry is sophisticated jewelry like necklaces, rings, bracelets, and some fashionable and trendy watches, like others, are embedded in small devices that can notify and track events.

Modern smart jewelry includes; Altruist, Bellabeat LEAF for stress tracking, Shine by Misfit Swarovski; activity monitor and sleep monitor, Ear-O-Smart; earrings that measure activity, calories, and heart rate, Arc pendants for men; used by cyclists for road navigation, MICA Opening Ceremonies, Tory Burch & Fitbit, Ringly and many more.

Implant Device

These are devices that are implanted under the skin primarily for medical reasons, such as insulin pumps, retinal implants, magnetic sensors, smart drugs, etc. Many proponents believe that these implantable devices could become part of the human body in the near future.

How safe is this wearable technology?

There has been much controversy about the potential health hazards of these wearables. It is a well-known fact that some mobile phones with low radiation can cause several health problems, moreover electronic devices that are carried very close to the body for a long time will not cause more serious harm to the user.

Most researchers have confirmed this fact, while some have disproved it with extensive research to prove their point. However, a group from the World Health Organization

(WHO) confirmed in a recent 2011 study that there is a possibility that mobile devices that use radio waves can cause health problems and it is best to keep them away from the body to avoid this possibility.

With that in mind, why then do we have the invention of wearable devices placed on the body? If cell phones are likely to be hazardous to health, it's also possible that wearable technology could cause more harm because they carry the same electronic radiation as cell phones.

However, there are as many benefits to be derived from this wearable technology as seen before and since most wearable technologies use Bluetooth and Bluetooth uses less radio waves wearable technology is much safer than cell phones.

Chapter 4 - Advantages of using technology over not using it

Wearable devices are used in so many industries that their uses range from being able to save lives to monitoring the performance of basketball players in live games. Below is a brief summary of how the pros outweigh the cons when it comes to using wearables in various fields:

medical

FDA-approved medical-grade wearable devices provide patients with a non-intrusive way to monitor vital signs and a variety of health conditions. For example, a "smart pill" released by Proteus Digital Health monitors whether a person has taken their medication for the day, which can mean a life-or-death situation for seniors with memory problems. There are other similar tools for pain management, diabetes, heart health, and more.

communication and security

Wearables can go beyond instant messaging and connecting with people on social media. Wearing a tracking device that looks like a regular bracelet or watch can help locate missing children or loved ones with memory problems. Some gadgets are also equipped with a one-touch emergency call, which is indispensable in case of an emergency.

sports and health

Gone are the days when fitness trackers were just fancy pedometers. Today's wearable fitness equipment is so advanced that it can monitor vital signs in real-time, determine sleep quality, and correct poor posture - all contributing to good health.

In sports, wearable technology devices can act as virtual trainers and enhance athlete performance by monitoring every movement during training.

WHETHER FOR HEALTH or athletic performance, wearables provide personalized information that coaches, doctors, nutritionists, and other healthcare professionals can monitor.

company

In the corporate world, the use of wearables at work has increased productivity, engagement, and collaboration among employees. While security issues can be a concern for wearable technology, they can be resolved by ensuring that every device used for business has a cloud-based security solution.

lifestyle computer

Game worlds will never be the same with the return of virtual reality and immersive VR systems like the Virtuix Omni™, which consists of a gun, belt, VR headset, and platform. Among his many other groundbreaking inventions are Razor's open-source VR, Sony's Project Morpheus designed specifically for the PlayStation 4, and the Tesla suit.

Chapter 5 - Things to consider before investing

Just as you wouldn't go out and buy the first phone you come across without doing your research, you shouldn't go out and buy the first fitness device you come across just because you like it, or something to consider before you invest. in wearable fitness devices...

Price

Even though many tech brands are trying to lower the price of their devices, the majority of consumers are still unwilling to invest in a $300+ device. Decide how much you want to spend on a particular device. Of course, price usually aligns with how useful the gadget is for your particular situation. Will he be able to save your life? Can it help you lose weight? Will it organize your daily tasks? Can it simplify communication?

make and model

Many wearables fall into the "fitness tracker" category, but each offers different features. For example, the FitBit Charge HR is known for its heart rate monitoring, while the Jawbone UP3 has one of the best sleep-tracking features of any device today. If you take a look at the FitBit Alta, this sleek bracelet-like device only has basic fitness tracking capabilities without heart rate monitoring.

Design/Portability

Design is an important factor as you will be using most of these gadgets on a daily basis. In general, wearables should be comfortable. Most fitness clothing such as watches are made of some type of rubber and have a strap or buckle to adjust the band. Others are designed to look like regular watches, jewelry, or bracelets.

Battery life

It is important to determine how long a portable device can operate before it needs to be recharged. This is especially important if you are running long distances or hiking. Keep in mind that maintaining your device's battery can be a chore in the long run. Do you want to add another daily charger device to your smartphone, tablet, laptop, etc.? Fitness trackers like the Fitbit Zip (up to 6 months) and Garmin Vivofit (over a year) often last for months, while smartwatches like the Samsung Gear can last up to 24 hours.

data security

One of the most important things to consider is how secure your personal information is after connecting your device to a third-party website or app. Brands are fully responsible for the security of any personal information you provide. Hence, it is best to choose a popular brand that is known for always testing its products.

Compatibility with other devices

FITNESS OF THE FUTURE: GETTING STARTED WITH FITNESS TECHNOLOGY

Determine if the wearable you want to buy is compatible with your existing device. In general, the Apple Watch requires an iPhone 5 or later, whereas Android-based smartwatches will not work on any iPhone. Want to replace some of your existing devices with wearables?

These 6 key considerations will help you decide whether a wearable is right for your situation or ensure you buy the best one that fits your needs.

Determine if the wearable you want to buy is compatible with your existing device. In general, the Apple Watch requires an iPhone 5 or later, whereas Android-based smartwatches will not work on an iPhone. Want to replace some of your existing devices with wearables?

These 6 key considerations will help you decide whether a wearable is right for your situation or ensure you buy the best one that fits your needs.

Chapter 6 - A comparison of wearable technologies and smartphone applications

One of the most frequently asked questions about wearable technology is:

What can it offer that a multi-app smartphone can't?

This is a perfectly normal question because buying a new device that simply duplicates the features of your existing one seems like a waste of investment.

In a 2015 trial published in the Journal of the American Medical Association, six of the most popular fitness trackers showed they provided the same results as the four best smartphone fitness apps. However, this research only focuses on the pedometer functions of wearable devices and applications.

The sleep-tracking wearable works in a similar way to a smartphone with a sleep-tracking app. The user must press a button to "tell" the device to go to sleep. The advantage of wearable technology is that it provides more information, such as sleep quality (Fatigue Science), dreams (Luciding), or sleep waves and muscle tension during sleep (Neuro: On).

In healthcare, there are no smartphone apps that help track users' glucose levels (Google Verily Glass), pain management (Quell Relief and Cur), nausea (ReliefBand), asthma (Health Care

Originals Intelligent Asthma Management), back problems (UPRIGHT and Lumo). lifts), low back muscle pain (Valedo), and other specific health conditions.

There are many wearable technology devices designed for athletic performance that smartphone apps can't beat. For example, the vest-like slingshot is used by many NFL teams to monitor an athlete's heart rate, pace, and more than 100 other metrics to help prevent injury during practice or games. Used by NBA players, the Athos three-piece set is designed to monitor muscle, breathing, and heart rate data in real time.

In other cases, the wearable and the smartphone app are used together to create a unique system. Ford's plant in Valencia, Spain, is the first to adapt its wearable quality assurance device, a wrist-worn smartphone-like device, as part of its daily QA tasks. Operated by a smartphone app, it saves 1 kilometer of a worker walking each day by completely eliminating production line paper systems.

Comparing wearable technology and smartphone apps is difficult because both can benefit the user. The great thing is that with the advent of wearables, smartphone companies are trying to step up their game and include built-in features that match wearable technology. On the other hand, wearable tech brands think outside the box to meet needs that smartphone apps can't match. In hindsight, it's a win-win for consumers whether they opt for a wearable or stick with their smartphone app.

Chapter 7 - Avoiding Common Wearable Technology Newbie Mistakes

Wearable technology goes beyond fitness trackers. This technology has been adapted to a wide range of applications across a wide range of industries, from IT to fashion, sports to security, communications to medicine, and many more. Below are the 7 most common rookie mistakes users make when it comes to wearable technology:

Do not enter any personal information

Wearables often provide users with online accounts or access to applications where data can be monitored. While sharing personal information can be difficult for anyone concerned with security, adding your own information will actually help maximize the potential of your device. This is especially true for fitness trackers with advanced features like calories burned/calories burned, as weight, height, and other vitals are calculated along with the new metrics.

Expect all wearables to be 100% accurate

Not all wearables are the same. For example, a medical fitness tracker may be able to provide 100% accurate results, but other non-FDA-approved trackers may have accuracy issues. The key to finding devices with good data accuracy is to check which devices have been tested, validated, or certified by a third-party organization, such as a university or testing laboratory.

Does not set up or calibrate the device

Although most manufacturers inform users that calibrating the device is optional, some wearable data inaccuracies can be resolved by simply checking the device settings.

You don't research

This is one of the biggest mistakes.

Imagine this scenario - a person decides to change his lifestyle and become more active. To do that, they might want to grab one of those neat gadgets that let you track calories burned, steps taken, heart rate, and all that neat stuff. They don't know what they are doing, they just know they want it. So with that in mind, they went out and bought the first thing they came across.

Therein lies one of the mistakes that you should avoid. Never go out and buy wearable tech before you've done your research. If you do your research, you need to find out about features, data, battery, and all nine meters.

Ask a sales representative

You shouldn't ask a sales rep what's the best. They will most likely give you the wrong advice and guide you on what to buy.

Set unrealistic goals

FITNESS OF THE FUTURE: GETTING STARTED WITH FITNESS TECHNOLOGY

Whether you're looking for workout clothes that can potentially help you lose weight or devices that can streamline your daily communications, it's important to set realistic goals.

In the end, these gadgets are just gadgets. If you're trying to lose weight, you should still be trying and not just relying on your device. If you want to reduce the number of devices you use for social media, email, and other tasks, it's up to you whether you stick with smartwatches or other types of wearable technology. Of course, this does not apply to wearable medical devices and implantable materials designed to prevent pain, treat disease, or even save lives.

Confusing term "water resistant"

With fitness trackers, manufacturers often indicate whether the device is waterproof. However, this is difficult to interpret as some devices will get wet but will be damaged if submerged in water. Other devices are specifically designed for use while bathing or swimming. It is important to determine how well the device works underwater or not at all.

These 7 common mistakes can be avoided by doing thorough research before purchasing any portable device. Avoiding these mistakes not only allows the user to maximize the potential of the device, but also extends the life of the wearable technology.

Chapter 8 – Integrating wearable technology into everyday life

So many people buy wearable technology devices with the idea of changing their lives. They use it for two days, maybe even two weeks before they shove it in the bottom of the drawer and forget about it altogether. Do you want to do that? Of course not.

Once you buy a device, you want to use it every day for as long as possible. After all, it's a device designed to help you get your life back, right? So what's the use in the bottom of your drawer? They must learn to make wearable technology a part of everyday life.

get used to it

This kind of custom here is good - you have to get used to wearable technology. Think about it, when you first got your phone, have you ever accidentally dropped it? Now you may never imagine yourself without this phone by your side. If you are used to using these portable devices, there will come a time when you cannot imagine yourself without them.

Set goals and stick to them

Set a goal to make wearables a part of your everyday life and stick to that goal. If you've decided that a wearable device can make your life a lot easier, it can become as much a part of your everyday life as a smartphone.

Tips on how to make fitness a part of your life

A fitness tracker with sleep monitoring, pedometer, and heart rate capabilities can be your motivation for a big lifestyle change. By turning the sleep feature on and off every time you go to bed and wake up, you can follow a much healthier sleep pattern through the sleep data you record. With the pedometer function, you can see if you take more than 10,000 steps per day, which is the recommended daily activity for everyone to follow.

For wearable medical devices to monitor health problems, their integration into everyday life is critical. If you have a cardiovascular condition that requires regular monitoring, be sure to wear the device on your chest (Polar H7), as a patch (Monika Novii System or Zio XT patch), on your body (FitLinxx AmpStrip), on your hip (LEO), on your head (Imec EEG Headset) or other body parts, every time you wake up or before doing physical activity.

Sports fans can get inside information about the matches they watch live. With sports leagues connecting to wearables, connecting/pinning athletes to devices during gameplay, and collaborating with technology companies to create new experiences, people at home can view comprehensive player stats during gameplay.

Smartwatches and trackers such as bracelets allow users to check email, make/answer calls, view social media notifications, and stream other communications with just one device. However,

FITNESS OF THE FUTURE: GETTING STARTED WITH FITNESS TECHNOLOGY

like smartphones, how a user uses wearable features can determine whether a device is an effective addition to everyday life or simply a "diversion".

Conclusion - The future of wearable technology: where did it come from here?

Well, we've reached the top of our wearables for beginners guide, and I want to congratulate you on getting this far. In this last section, we look to the future and what's next for wearable technology.

Software has dominated the technology industry for over 15 years. With smartphones being embraced by everyone around the world since the mid-2000s, hardware is definitely making a comeback and isn't going to die anytime soon.

Today we are seeing the emergence of exciting devices such as drones, connected homes, wearable technology, and other devices that are considered part of the Internet of Things (IoT). This IoT is a physical object that is equipped with sensors, software, electronics, various types of technology, or network connectivity that allows objects to collect, record, and share data.

The future of wearable healthcare technology is as exciting as it is frightening. In the medical field, manufacturers are testing mood-monitoring devices and neurocentric wearables that use brain stimulation to treat pain at home. Implantable devices, in which a small device is implanted in the user's body, can be a life-saving device, but users are still skeptical not only about the cost but also about the device's invasion.

In business, companies will continue to find applications for wearables that will enhance employee collaboration and productivity. Advertisers will also find ways for ad placement in mobile device apps.

More and more wearable devices are being developed to address business operations (logistics, customer service), communications (social media, multimedia), security (emergency services, ambulance tracking), health and well-being (obesity management, non-intrusive patient monitoring). Sports (training, performance tracking), fashion (reactive reactions), games (HUD, VR, augmented reality), and other areas.

2016 may seem like a peak year for the wearables industry, but as the upcoming product announcements at the last CES proved, wearables are here to stay.

Also by J. Steele

Gemstone Guide Book: A Simple Informative Handbook
Born to Win: Discover Unlimited Possibilities
Think You Can and You Will: How to Become a Champion in Life
Quick and Easy Guide on Dieting
Quick and Easy Guide on Fashion
Alcohol and Addictions
Online Dating
Lose Weight Dieting
Lose Weight Fasting
Ways To Lose Weight For Women
Raw Food and Healthy Living
Back Pain Recovery Informative Guide
100 Health Suggestions: A Healthy Lifestyle is Beneficial to the Soul
Tips for Bodybuilding
Vegetarianism's Advantages
Fitness of the Future: Getting Started With Fitness Technology
The Shadow's Blade: A Tale of Magic and Betrayal

About the Publisher

Accepting manuscripts in the most categories. We love to help people get their words available to the world.

Revival Waves of Glory focus is to provide more options to be published. We do traditional paperbacks, hardcovers, audio books and ebooks all over the world. A traditional royalty-based publisher that offers self-publishing options, Revival Waves provides a very author friendly and transparent publishing process, with President Bill Vincent involved in the full process of your book. Send us your manuscript and we will contact you as soon as possible.

Contact: Bill Vincent at rwgpublishing@yahoo.com